Table Of Contents

Chapter 1: Introduction to Physical Fitness and Exercise

The Importance of Physical Fitness in Adulthood

Physical fitness is a crucial aspect of leading a healthy and fulfilling life, especially in adulthood. As we age, our bodies naturally go through various changes, and maintaining a regular exercise routine becomes even more essential. In this subchapter, we will explore the significance of physical fitness in adulthood and how it can positively impact our overall well-being.

Regular exercise in adulthood offers numerous benefits that extend beyond just physical health. Engaging in physical activity helps improve cardiovascular health, strengthens muscles and bones, and enhances flexibility and balance. These benefits are particularly important as we age since they can help prevent chronic diseases such as heart disease, diabetes, and osteoporosis. By incorporating regular exercise into our daily routine, we can significantly reduce the risk of developing these conditions and improve our overall quality of life.

Moreover, physical fitness plays a vital role in maintaining a healthy weight and preventing weight-related issues. As we age, our metabolism tends to slow down, making it easier to gain weight. Regular exercise helps to boost metabolism, burn calories, and build lean muscle mass, thus aiding in weight management. Additionally, exercise stimulates the release of endorphins, which are natural mood enhancers. This can help alleviate stress, reduce anxiety, and combat depression, ultimately leading to a better mental and emotional well-being.

In order to achieve optimal physical fitness in adulthood, it is crucial to adopt a holistic approach that combines regular exercise with a balanced and nutritious diet. Proper nutrition is essential to fuel our bodies and provide the necessary nutrients for energy, muscle repair, and overall well-being. By incorporating whole foods, including fruits, vegetables, lean proteins, and whole grains, we can ensure that our bodies receive the necessary vitamins and minerals to support our fitness goals.

In conclusion, physical fitness is of utmost importance in adulthood, benefiting not only our physical health but also our mental and emotional well-being. Regular exercise helps prevent chronic diseases, maintain a healthy weight, and improve overall quality of life. When combined with a balanced diet, physical fitness becomes even more effective in promoting a healthy lifestyle. By prioritizing our physical fitness, we can lead a fulfilling and vibrant life well into adulthood.

Benefits of Regular Exercise for Adults

Regular exercise is not only beneficial for your physical health but also plays a key role in promoting mental well-being and overall quality of life. This chapter explores the numerous advantages that adults can gain from incorporating regular exercise into their daily routines.

1. Improved Physical Fitness: Engaging in regular exercise helps improve cardiovascular health, strengthens muscles and bones, and enhances flexibility and endurance. Physical fitness allows adults to perform daily activities with ease, maintain independence, and reduce the risk of chronic diseases such as heart disease, diabetes, and obesity.

2. Weight Management: Regular exercise is essential for weight loss and weight maintenance. It helps burn calories and build muscle mass, which increases metabolism and aids in shedding excess weight. Combined with a healthy diet, exercise promotes a sustainable and healthy weight loss journey for adults.

3. Mental Well-being: Exercise is a powerful mood booster and stress reliever. It stimulates the release of endorphins, also known as "feel-good" hormones, which help reduce symptoms of anxiety, depression, and stress. Regular exercise can improve cognitive function, memory, and overall mental clarity, enabling adults to lead a happier and more fulfilling life.

4. Enhanced Energy Levels: Engaging in physical activity regularly increases energy levels and combats fatigue. Exercise improves blood circulation, delivering oxygen and nutrients to the body's tissues, which helps increase energy levels and improve focus and productivity throughout the day.

5. Disease Prevention: Regular exercise is a vital component in preventing various chronic diseases. It helps manage blood pressure, control blood sugar levels, reduce the risk of heart disease, stroke, and certain types of cancer. Exercise also strengthens the immune system, reducing susceptibility to illnesses and infections.

6. Improved Sleep Quality: Regular exercise promotes better sleep patterns and quality. Physical activity helps regulate sleep-wake cycles, reduces insomnia, and improves overall sleep duration and quality. Adults who exercise regularly experience deeper and more restful sleep, waking up feeling refreshed and rejuvenated.

7. Enhanced Longevity: Research consistently shows that regular exercise is linked to increased life expectancy. Engaging in physical activity reduces the risk of premature death and age-related decline, allowing adults to maintain optimal health and vitality as they age.

To reap these benefits, incorporate at least 150 minutes of moderate-intensity aerobic exercise or 75 minutes of vigorous-intensity exercise into your weekly routine. Remember to consult with a healthcare professional before starting any new exercise program to ensure it aligns with your current health status and abilities. Start small, set achievable goals, and gradually increase the duration and intensity of your workouts. Remember, consistency is key to unlocking the full potential of regular exercise for your physical fitness, mental well-being, and overall health.

Common Barriers to Exercise and How to Overcome Them

Introduction:
In our fast-paced lives, finding time and motivation to exercise regularly can be challenging. However, understanding and overcoming common barriers to exercise is crucial for achieving optimal physical fitness and overall well-being. In this subchapter, we will explore some of the most prevalent obstacles adults face when trying to incorporate exercise into their lives. Moreover, we will provide practical strategies to overcome these barriers, enabling you to lead a healthy and active lifestyle.

1. Lack of Time:

One of the most common barriers to exercise for adults is a perceived lack of time. With work, family obligations, and other responsibilities, finding a spare moment for physical activity may seem impossible. However, it's essential to prioritize your health. Consider incorporating short bursts of exercise throughout your day, such as taking the stairs instead of the elevator or going for a brisk walk during your lunch break. Additionally, planning your exercise routine in advance and scheduling it into your calendar can help you adhere to your fitness goals.

2. Lack of Motivation:

Finding the motivation to exercise regularly can be challenging, especially when faced with competing priorities. To overcome this barrier, identify your personal fitness goals and remind yourself of the numerous benefits exercise offers, including increased energy, improved mood, and better overall health. Consider joining group fitness classes or finding a workout buddy to keep you accountable and motivated. Experiment with different forms of exercise until you find activities that you genuinely enjoy, making it easier to maintain your enthusiasm.

3. Fear of Injury:

Many adults worry about the risk of injury when engaging in physical activity. However, taking proper precautions can significantly reduce this risk. Start slowly and gradually increase the intensity and duration of your workouts. Always warm up before exercising and cool down afterward. If you are unsure about proper form or technique, seek guidance from a qualified fitness professional. Additionally, wearing appropriate footwear and using protective equipment, if necessary, can enhance your safety during exercise.

4. Lack of Support:

Having a strong support system can make a significant difference in your exercise journey. Communicate your fitness goals to your family and friends, and ask for their support. Consider joining fitness communities or online groups where you can connect with like-minded individuals who share similar objectives. Surrounding yourself with positive and encouraging people can provide the necessary motivation and accountability to overcome barriers and achieve your exercise goals.

Conclusion:
While barriers to exercise may vary for adults, it is important to recognize and address them to lead a healthy and active lifestyle. By acknowledging common obstacles such as lack of time, motivation, fear of injury, and lack of support, you can develop strategies to overcome them. Remember, making exercise a priority and incorporating it into your daily routine will not only benefit your physical fitness but also your mental well-being. With determination, planning, and support, you can overcome these barriers and embark on a fulfilling journey towards optimal health and wellness.

Chapter 2: Understanding Physical Fitness Components

Cardiovascular Endurance

In the pursuit of physical fitness and overall health, one cannot overlook the importance of cardiovascular endurance. This subchapter aims to shed light on the significance of cardiovascular endurance for adults, providing valuable insights into how it can be improved through exercise, nutrition, and a healthy lifestyle.

Cardiovascular endurance refers to the ability of the heart, lungs, and blood vessels to deliver oxygen and nutrients to the working muscles efficiently. It is a key component of fitness and plays a vital role in maintaining a healthy body weight, reducing the risk of chronic diseases, and promoting overall well-being.

Regular exercise is crucial for enhancing cardiovascular endurance. Engaging in activities such as running, swimming, cycling, or brisk walking can help strengthen the heart muscle, increase lung capacity, and improve oxygen utilization. It is recommended that adults aim for at least 150 minutes of moderate-intensity aerobic exercise or 75 minutes of vigorous-intensity aerobic exercise each week. Incorporating a variety of exercises and gradually increasing the intensity and duration will yield optimal results.

In addition to exercise, nutrition plays a pivotal role in improving cardiovascular endurance. A diet rich in fruits, vegetables, whole grains, lean proteins, and healthy fats can provide the necessary nutrients to support cardiovascular health. Consuming foods high in antioxidants, such as berries, dark leafy greens, and nuts, can help fight inflammation and protect against heart disease. Moreover, reducing the intake of saturated and trans fats, sodium, and added sugars is crucial for maintaining optimal heart health.

Adopting a healthy lifestyle is equally important in improving cardiovascular endurance. Avoiding tobacco use and excessive alcohol consumption are vital steps to protect the heart and blood vessels. Managing stress through techniques like meditation, yoga, or deep breathing exercises can also positively impact cardiovascular health. Additionally, ensuring an adequate amount of quality sleep is essential for the body's recovery and rejuvenation, further supporting cardiovascular function.

By focusing on improving cardiovascular endurance through exercise, nutrition, and a healthy lifestyle, adults can experience numerous benefits. These include increased energy levels, improved mood, enhanced weight management, and reduced risk of heart disease, stroke, and other chronic conditions.

In conclusion, cardiovascular endurance is a critical aspect of physical fitness and overall health for adults. Incorporating regular exercise, following a nutritious diet, and adopting a healthy lifestyle are key strategies to enhance cardiovascular endurance. By prioritizing these elements, adults can pave the way towards a fit, healthy, and vibrant life.

Muscular Strength and Endurance

Building and maintaining muscular strength and endurance are crucial components of a well-rounded fitness regimen. In this subchapter, we will delve into the importance of these attributes, as well as provide practical tips and exercises to help you enhance your muscular strength and endurance.

Muscular strength refers to the ability of your muscles to exert maximum force against resistance. This type of strength is vital for performing daily activities, such as lifting heavy objects or pushing a car. By incorporating strength training exercises into your routine, you can increase your lean muscle mass, improve your overall strength, and enhance your metabolism.

Endurance, on the other hand, is the ability of your muscles to sustain repetitive contractions over an extended period. Endurance exercises are essential for improving cardiovascular health, increasing stamina, and enhancing overall performance. Regular endurance training can also contribute to weight loss by burning calories and boosting your metabolism.

To develop muscular strength, it is recommended to engage in resistance training exercises at least two to three times a week. This can include weightlifting, bodyweight exercises, or using resistance bands. Start with lighter weights and gradually increase the resistance as your muscles adapt and become stronger. Remember to maintain proper form and technique to prevent injuries.

To improve muscular endurance, consider incorporating activities such as running, swimming, cycling, or high-intensity interval training (HIIT) into your fitness routine. These exercises challenge your muscles to work for an extended period, strengthening them and enhancing their endurance capacity. Aim for at least 150 minutes of moderate-intensity endurance training or 75 minutes of vigorous-intensity training per week.

In addition to exercise, proper nutrition plays a vital role in developing muscular strength and endurance. Ensure that your diet includes an adequate amount of protein, which is essential for muscle repair and growth. Incorporate a variety of fruits, vegetables, whole grains, and lean proteins into your meals to fuel your workouts and promote optimal muscle function.

By prioritizing muscular strength and endurance in your fitness journey, you can experience numerous benefits, including increased energy levels, improved overall health, enhanced athletic performance, and weight management. Remember to consult with a healthcare professional before starting any new exercise program, especially if you have any underlying health conditions.

In conclusion, muscular strength and endurance are fundamental aspects of physical fitness. By incorporating regular strength and endurance training exercises into your routine, alongside a balanced diet, you can achieve optimal health and well-being.

Body Composition

Understanding your body composition is a crucial aspect of achieving overall physical fitness and maintaining a healthy lifestyle. It refers to the ratio of different types of tissues that make up your body, such as fat, muscle, bone, and water. In the book "Fit for Life: The Ultimate Guide to Physical Fitness and Exercise for Adults," we will delve into the significance of body composition and how it can impact your physical fitness, nutrition, and weight loss goals.

One of the key components of body composition is body fat percentage. While some amount of body fat is essential for insulation and energy storage, excessive fat can lead to various health issues, including heart disease and diabetes. This book will provide you with practical tips and strategies to reduce body fat through a combination of exercise and healthy eating habits. We will explore different types of exercises that can help you burn fat effectively, such as cardiovascular exercises, strength training, and high-intensity interval training (HIIT).

Furthermore, we will emphasize the importance of building and maintaining lean muscle mass. Muscle not only enhances your physical strength and endurance but also plays a vital role in increasing your metabolic rate. This means that having more muscle can help you burn calories more efficiently, even at rest. Our book will guide you on how to incorporate strength training exercises into your fitness routine to build lean muscle and improve your body composition.

Additionally, we will address the significance of proper nutrition in achieving an optimal body composition. A balanced diet that includes adequate protein, healthy fats, and complex carbohydrates is essential for supporting muscle growth, reducing body fat, and promoting overall health. We will provide you with practical nutrition advice and meal plans that align with your fitness goals and help you maintain a healthy body composition.

Whether you are aiming to lose weight, improve your physical fitness, or simply lead a healthier lifestyle, understanding and optimizing your body composition is crucial. By following the guidance and recommendations in this book, you will gain the knowledge and tools necessary to achieve your desired body composition and unlock your full potential for physical fitness and overall well-being. Get ready to embark on a transformative journey towards a healthier, fitter, and happier you.

Chapter 3: Creating a Personalized Fitness Plan

Assessing Your Current Fitness Level

Before embarking on any fitness journey, it is crucial to assess your current fitness level. This assessment will not only provide you with a baseline to measure your progress but also help you tailor your exercise and nutrition plan to your specific needs and goals. In this chapter, we will explore various methods to assess your current fitness level and provide you with the tools to get started on your journey towards a healthier and fitter lifestyle.

One of the simplest ways to assess your current fitness level is by evaluating your overall physical activity. Consider your daily routine and the amount of time you spend engaging in physical activities such as walking, jogging, or participating in sports. Are you leading a sedentary lifestyle or incorporating regular physical activity into your routine? This self-reflection will help you determine the starting point of your fitness journey.

Next, let's evaluate your cardiovascular endurance. This is an essential component of fitness and reflects your ability to sustain aerobic activities over a period of time. You can assess your cardiovascular endurance by performing a simple test such as walking or jogging for a specific distance or time and monitoring your heart rate and breathing patterns. This will give you an idea of your current cardiovascular fitness level and help you set realistic goals for improvement.

Strength and muscular endurance are also important aspects of fitness. Assessing your current strength levels can be done through basic exercises such as push-ups, squats, or planks. Take note of how many repetitions you can perform and the level of resistance you can handle. This will help you design a strength training program tailored to your abilities.

Additionally, evaluating your flexibility is crucial to overall fitness. Assessing your flexibility can be as simple as performing basic stretches and noting any limitations or discomfort you experience. Flexibility exercises are vital for injury prevention and maintaining proper posture.

Finally, consider your body composition. This refers to the ratio of fat mass to lean muscle mass in your body. Assessing your body composition can be done through various methods such as skinfold measurements or bioelectrical impedance analysis. Knowing your body composition will help you set realistic weight loss or muscle gain goals and track your progress accurately.

By assessing your current fitness level, you will gain valuable insights into your strengths and weaknesses. Armed with this knowledge, you can develop a personalized fitness and nutrition plan that will help you achieve your goals effectively. Remember, everyone's starting point is different, and progress is the key.

Setting Realistic Goals

In the journey towards achieving physical fitness and leading a healthy lifestyle, setting realistic goals is crucial. Without clear objectives in mind, it's easy to become overwhelmed or discouraged, leading to a lack of motivation and ultimately giving up on your fitness and nutrition journey. This subchapter of "Fit for Life: The Ultimate Guide to Physical Fitness and Exercise for Adults" aims to guide adults in setting realistic goals that are attainable and sustainable, ultimately leading to long-term success in physical fitness, nutrition, and weight loss.

When it comes to setting goals, it's important to be specific and measurable. Instead of vague goals like "I want to get fit," consider specific objectives like "I want to be able to run a 5K in under 30 minutes within three months." This allows you to track your progress and celebrate small victories along the way. It's also essential to set realistic timelines for your goals, ensuring that they are achievable within a reasonable timeframe.

Another crucial aspect of goal setting is to make them personal and meaningful to you. Your goals should align with your individual interests and motivations. For example, if you enjoy swimming, your goal could be to swim a certain number of laps or participate in a swim meet. By making your goals personally relevant, you are more likely to stay committed and motivated throughout your journey.

It's also important to set both short-term and long-term goals. Short-term goals allow you to focus on smaller milestones that lead to your ultimate objective. For instance, if your long-term goal is to lose 50 pounds, your short-term goals could be to lose 2 pounds per week or to exercise for at least 30 minutes daily. These smaller achievements will keep you motivated and provide a sense of accomplishment.

In addition to setting goals related to physical fitness and exercise, it's important to integrate nutrition and healthy eating into your objectives. Consider setting goals such as incorporating more fruits and vegetables into your daily meals, reducing your intake of processed foods, or cooking at home more often. By combining exercise and healthy eating goals, you create a holistic approach to your overall well-being.

Remember, setting realistic goals is not about perfection. It's about progress and consistency. Be flexible and adjust your goals as needed. Celebrate your achievements, no matter how small, and learn from any setbacks. By setting realistic goals that are tailored to your interests and motivations, you are setting yourself up for success on your journey towards physical fitness, nutrition, weight loss, and a healthy lifestyle.

Designing an Effective Exercise Program

When it comes to achieving optimal physical fitness and leading a healthy lifestyle, designing an effective exercise program is paramount. A well-designed program not only helps you achieve your fitness goals but also ensures you stay motivated and committed to your exercise routine. In this subchapter, we will explore the key components of designing an effective exercise program that is tailored to the needs of adults.

1. Set Clear Goals: Before starting any exercise program, it is essential to set clear and achievable goals. Whether your aim is to lose weight, improve cardiovascular health, build strength, or enhance flexibility, having a specific goal in mind will help you structure your program accordingly.

2. Assess Your Fitness Level: Understanding your current fitness level is crucial in designing an effective exercise program. Assess your cardiovascular endurance, muscular strength, flexibility, and body composition to determine where you stand. This assessment will serve as a baseline to track your progress and make necessary adjustments to your program.

3. Choose the Right Exercises: Select exercises that target different muscle groups and accommodate your fitness level. Including a mix of cardiovascular exercises like walking, jogging, or cycling, along with strength training exercises using resistance bands or weights, will provide a well-rounded workout routine. Don't forget to incorporate exercises that improve flexibility, such as yoga or stretching exercises.

4. Create a Balanced Routine: It is crucial to strike a balance between cardiovascular exercises, strength training, and flexibility exercises. Aim for at least 150 minutes of moderate-intensity aerobic activity or 75 minutes of vigorous-intensity aerobic activity per week. Additionally, include strength training exercises at least twice a week, targeting major muscle groups.

5. Consider Personal Preferences: Design an exercise program that aligns with your personal preferences. If you enjoy group activities, consider joining fitness classes or sports clubs. If you prefer solitude, opt for activities like swimming or hiking. By incorporating activities you enjoy, you are more likely to stick to your program in the long run.

6. Gradually Increase Intensity: As your fitness level improves, gradually increase the intensity and duration of your workouts. This progressive overload helps you avoid plateaus and continue making progress towards your fitness goals.

7. Listen to Your Body: Pay attention to your body's cues and adjust your exercise program accordingly. If you experience pain or discomfort, modify or seek professional guidance. Remember, exercise should challenge you but not cause harm.

Designing an effective exercise program is the foundation for a healthy lifestyle. By setting clear goals, assessing your fitness level, choosing the right exercises, creating a balanced routine, considering personal preferences, gradually increasing intensity, and listening to your body, you can create a program that suits your needs and helps you achieve optimal physical fitness and overall well-being.

Incorporating Variety and Progression in Your Routine

One of the keys to achieving optimal physical fitness and maintaining a healthy lifestyle is to incorporate variety and progression into your exercise routine. By doing so, you not only keep yourself motivated and engaged but also continue to challenge your body, allowing for greater gains in strength, endurance, and overall fitness.

When it comes to physical fitness and exercise, variety is the spice of life. Performing the same exercises day in and day out can quickly become monotonous and lead to boredom or a plateau in your progress. By incorporating different types of exercises, such as cardiovascular activities, strength training, and flexibility exercises, you can target different muscle groups and improve your overall fitness level.

Furthermore, adding variety to your routine can also prevent overuse injuries that may occur from repetitive movements. By engaging in various activities, you not only reduce the risk of injury but also enhance your overall physical capabilities. Consider trying new fitness classes, outdoor activities, or sports to keep your workouts fresh and exciting.

In addition to variety, progression is crucial for continued improvement. Your body is an amazing machine that adapts to the stress you place upon it. By gradually increasing the intensity, duration, or frequency of your workouts, you can challenge your body to continually improve. This progression can be achieved by adding more weight, increasing the number of repetitions or sets, or incorporating interval training.

Progression not only helps you reach your fitness goals but also prevents plateaus. When you challenge your body, it responds by growing stronger and fitter. Without progression, your body becomes accustomed to the demands of your workouts and your progress may stagnate. Keep pushing yourself and striving for improvement to see the best results.

Remember, variety and progression are not limited to just exercise. Nutrition and healthy eating play a significant role in your overall fitness journey. Incorporate a variety of nutrient-dense foods into your diet to ensure you are getting all the essential vitamins, minerals, and macronutrients your body needs. Gradually make healthier food choices and consider portion control to support weight loss or maintenance.

By incorporating variety and progression into your routine, you can keep your workouts interesting, prevent plateaus, and achieve your fitness goals. Embrace new activities, challenge yourself, and make healthy food choices to become fit for life. Remember, it's never too late to start taking care of your physical fitness and overall health.

Chapter 4: Cardiovascular Exercise for Adults

Introduction to Cardiovascular Exercise

Cardiovascular exercise, also known as aerobic exercise, plays a crucial role in maintaining and improving physical fitness and overall health. In this subchapter, we will explore the benefits of cardiovascular exercise, the various forms it can take, and how to incorporate it into your daily routine.

Physical Fitness and Exercise:
Regular cardiovascular exercise is essential for achieving and maintaining optimal physical fitness. By engaging in activities that elevate your heart rate, you enhance your cardiovascular endurance, strengthen your heart and lungs, and improve your overall stamina. These exercises also help to lower blood pressure, reduce the risk of heart disease, and increase bone density.

Nutrition and Healthy Eating:
In conjunction with a balanced and nutritious diet, cardiovascular exercise is a key component in achieving and maintaining a healthy weight. Engaging in activities such as running, cycling, swimming, or dancing can help burn calories, boost metabolism, and promote weight loss. Additionally, cardiovascular exercise can improve insulin sensitivity, regulate blood sugar levels, and contribute to a healthy metabolism.

Weight Loss and Healthy Lifestyle:
Cardiovascular exercise is a powerful tool for individuals seeking to lose weight and adopt a healthier lifestyle. By combining regular aerobic activity with a balanced diet, you can create a calorie deficit and promote fat loss. Furthermore, engaging in cardiovascular exercise releases endorphins, which can improve mood, reduce stress, and enhance overall well-being.

Incorporating Cardiovascular Exercise into Your Routine:
There are numerous forms of cardiovascular exercise that can be tailored to fit your interests, fitness level, and lifestyle. Whether it's brisk walking, jogging, swimming, cycling, dancing, or participating in group fitness classes, the key is to find activities that you enjoy and can sustain over time. Aim for at least 150 minutes of moderate-intensity aerobic activity, or 75 minutes of vigorous-intensity aerobic activity, per week.

Remember to start slowly and gradually increase the intensity and duration of your workouts. Listen to your body and consult with a healthcare professional if you have any underlying health conditions or concerns. Additionally, don't forget to warm up before each session and cool down afterward to prevent injury and promote recovery.

In conclusion, cardiovascular exercise is a fundamental aspect of physical fitness, nutrition, weight loss, and a healthy lifestyle. By incorporating regular aerobic activity into your routine, you can enjoy the numerous benefits it offers, including improved cardiovascular health, weight management, and overall well-being. So lace-up your sneakers, find an activity you love, and start reaping the rewards of cardiovascular exercise today.

Choosing the Right Cardiovascular Activities

When it comes to physical fitness and exercise, cardiovascular activities play a vital role in promoting a healthy lifestyle. Engaging in these activities not only helps in weight loss but also improves overall cardiovascular health and enhances endurance. But with so many options available, how do you choose the right cardiovascular activities that suit your needs and preferences? Let's explore some key factors to consider when making this decision.

First and foremost, it's essential to select activities that you enjoy. Finding an exercise that you genuinely look forward to will make it easier to stick to your fitness routine. Whether it's jogging, swimming, dancing, cycling, or playing a sport, the more you enjoy the activity, the more likely you are to make it a regular part of your life.

Consider your current fitness level and any physical limitations you may have. If you are just starting, low-impact exercises like walking or using an elliptical machine may be more suitable. As you progress, you can gradually increase the intensity and duration of your workouts. If you have any health concerns or injuries, it's advisable to consult with a healthcare professional before beginning any new exercise program.

Another crucial factor to consider is the convenience and accessibility of the activity. Evaluate your schedule and determine what fits best into your daily routine. If you have limited time, activities like high-intensity interval training (HIIT) can provide a quick and efficient workout. On the other hand, if you prefer to exercise outdoors, options like running or hiking might be more appealing.

Variety is also key when choosing cardiovascular activities. Mixing up your workouts not only prevents boredom but also challenges different muscle groups and keeps your body guessing. Incorporating a combination of aerobic exercises, such as running or swimming, and anaerobic exercises, such as weightlifting or circuit training, can provide a well-rounded fitness routine.

Lastly, consider your long-term goals and aspirations. If weight loss is your primary objective, activities that burn a high number of calories, like running or kickboxing, may be ideal. However, if you aim to improve cardiovascular health or participate in a specific event, such as a marathon or a cycling race, you might want to focus on activities that enhance endurance and stamina.

In conclusion, selecting the right cardiovascular activities is crucial for achieving your fitness goals and maintaining a healthy lifestyle. By considering factors such as enjoyment, fitness level, convenience, variety, and long-term goals, you can find the perfect activities that suit your needs and keep you motivated on your fitness journey. Remember, consistency is key, so choose activities that you can commit to and make them a regular part of your daily routine. Get moving, stay active, and enjoy the numerous benefits that cardiovascular exercise brings to your life.

Guidelines for Safe and Effective Cardiovascular Training

Cardiovascular training plays a crucial role in achieving and maintaining optimal physical fitness. Not only does it improve cardiovascular health, but it also aids in weight loss, promotes overall well-being, and reduces the risk of chronic diseases. To ensure you are getting the most out of your cardiovascular workouts while keeping yourself safe, it is important to follow these guidelines:

1. Consult with a healthcare professional: Before embarking on any cardiovascular training program, it is advisable to consult with your healthcare provider, especially if you have any pre-existing medical conditions or concerns. They can provide valuable insights and guidance tailored to your specific needs.

2. Start gradually: If you are new to cardiovascular training or have been inactive for a while, it is essential to start slowly and gradually increase the intensity and duration of your workouts. This approach helps prevent injuries and allows your body to adapt to the increased demands over time.

3. Choose activities you enjoy: Engaging in cardiovascular exercises that you find enjoyable increases the likelihood of sticking to your routine. Options such as brisk walking, cycling, swimming, dancing, or playing a sport can make your workouts more fun and sustainable.

4. Warm-up and cool-down: Prior to starting any cardiovascular exercise, warm-up your muscles and prepare your body for the workout ahead. This can be done through light stretching or performing low-intensity exercises for 5-10 minutes. Similarly, after your workout, cool down by gradually reducing the intensity and incorporating stretching exercises to help prevent muscle soreness and promote flexibility.

5. Monitor your intensity: Pay attention to your heart rate during cardio workouts. A general rule of thumb is to aim for a target heart rate between 50-85% of your maximum heart rate. You can calculate this by subtracting your age from 220. Additionally, using a heart rate monitor or wearable fitness tracker can help you stay within your desired range.

6. Stay hydrated: Proper hydration is crucial during cardiovascular training. Drink water before, during, and after your workouts to prevent dehydration and maintain optimal performance.

By following these guidelines, you can ensure that your cardiovascular training is safe, effective, and enjoyable. Remember to listen to your body and make adjustments as needed. Regular cardiovascular exercise, along with a balanced diet and a healthy lifestyle, will help you achieve your fitness goals and lead a vibrant, active life.

Tracking Your Cardiovascular Progress

Monitoring and tracking your cardiovascular progress is an essential aspect of any fitness journey. Whether you are focusing on weight loss, improving your overall physical fitness, or adopting a healthier lifestyle, keeping tabs on your cardiovascular health can provide valuable insights into your progress and help you stay motivated.

One of the most effective ways to track your cardiovascular progress is by monitoring your heart rate during exercise. By wearing a heart rate monitor or using fitness trackers equipped with heart rate monitoring capabilities, you can keep track of your heart rate zones and ensure that you are working at an intensity that is suitable for your goals.

Tracking your heart rate can help you determine if you are pushing yourself too hard or not challenging yourself enough. By regularly monitoring your heart rate during different types of exercises, such as running, cycling, or swimming, you can identify trends and make adjustments to your workouts accordingly.

Another important metric to track is your endurance level. This can be measured by assessing how long you can sustain aerobic activities without feeling fatigued. Start by keeping a record of the duration of your workouts and gradually increase the time as your cardiovascular fitness improves. Not only will this help you track your progress, but it will also motivate you to keep pushing your limits.

In addition to monitoring your heart rate and endurance, tracking your recovery time after intense workouts is crucial. The time it takes for your heart rate to return to its resting state after exercise is a good indicator of your cardiovascular fitness. As you become fitter, you will notice that your recovery time shortens, indicating an improvement in your cardiovascular health.

Lastly, keeping a log of your exercise routine, including the type of activity, duration, and intensity, can provide a comprehensive overview of your cardiovascular progress. This log can serve as a reference point for evaluating your progress, identifying patterns, and making necessary adjustments to your workout routine.

Remember, tracking your cardiovascular progress is not only about achieving specific goals; it is about understanding your body and making informed decisions. By monitoring your heart rate, endurance, recovery time, and maintaining a detailed exercise log, you can stay on track towards a healthier and fitter lifestyle.

In the next chapter, we will delve into the importance of nutrition and healthy eating in supporting your cardiovascular progress.

Chapter 5: Strength Training for Adults

Benefits of Strength Training for Adults

Strength training, also known as resistance training, is an essential component of a well-rounded fitness routine. It involves exercises that build strength, endurance, and muscle mass by using resistance, such as weights or resistance bands. While many adults associate strength training with athletes or bodybuilders, it offers numerous benefits for individuals of all ages and fitness levels. In this subchapter, we will explore the benefits of strength training specifically tailored for adults.

One of the primary advantages of strength training is improved physical fitness. Regular strength training exercises help adults increase their muscle strength, which can enhance overall performance in daily activities. From lifting heavy groceries to climbing stairs with ease, having stronger muscles allows adults to maintain an active and independent lifestyle.

Additionally, strength training plays a crucial role in maintaining a healthy weight. As adults age, their metabolism tends to slow down, making weight management more challenging. Strength training can help combat this by increasing muscle mass, which in turn boosts metabolism and promotes fat burning. Incorporating strength training exercises into a comprehensive weight loss program can lead to more sustainable and long-lasting results.

Beyond physical fitness and weight management, strength training offers numerous health benefits. Regular strength training exercises have been shown to improve bone density, reducing the risk of osteoporosis and fractures. It also helps regulate blood sugar levels, making it an excellent strategy for individuals with diabetes or those at risk of developing it.

Additionally, strength training positively impacts mental health. Engaging in regular strength training can help reduce symptoms of anxiety and depression, boost self-confidence, and improve overall mood. The endorphins released during exercise contribute to a sense of well-being and relaxation, making strength training a powerful tool for stress management.

In conclusion, strength training is a vital component of any adult's fitness routine. Its benefits range from improved physical fitness and weight management to enhanced bone density and mental well-being. No matter your age or fitness level, incorporating strength training exercises into your routine can unlock a multitude of advantages that contribute to a healthier and more fulfilling lifestyle.

Different Types of Strength Training Exercises

Strength training is an integral part of any fitness routine. It not only helps in building muscles but also improves overall endurance, balance, and flexibility. In this subchapter, we will explore the different types of strength training exercises that can be incorporated into your fitness regimen.

1. Resistance Training: This type of strength training involves the use of external resistance, such as dumbbells, resistance bands, or weight machines. It targets specific muscle groups and helps in increasing muscle strength and size. Resistance training exercises can include bicep curls, bench press, squats, and lunges.

2. Bodyweight Exercises: These exercises use your own body weight as resistance. They are convenient and can be performed anywhere, without the need for any equipment. Examples of bodyweight exercises include push-ups, planks, squats, and burpees. They are excellent for improving overall strength and toning muscles.

3. Isometric Exercises: Isometric exercises involve contracting and holding a specific muscle or group of muscles without any joint movement. They are great for developing static strength and improving stability. Examples of isometric exercises include wall sits, planks, and static lunges.

4. Plyometric Exercises: Plyometric exercises are high-intensity movements that involve explosive muscle contractions. They help in improving power, speed, and overall athletic performance. Common plyometric exercises include box jumps, burpees, and medicine ball throws.

5. Circuit Training: Circuit training combines strength training exercises with cardiovascular exercises, providing a full-body workout. It involves performing a series of exercises with minimal rest in between. Circuit training is an efficient way to build strength, burn calories, and improve cardiovascular fitness.

6. CrossFit: CrossFit is a high-intensity training program that combines elements of weightlifting, cardio, and bodyweight exercises. It focuses on functional movements and aims to improve overall fitness and build strength. CrossFit workouts are known for their intensity and variety.

7. Resistance Bands: Resistance bands are versatile and portable, making them an excellent option for strength training exercises. They come in different resistance levels and can be used to target various muscle groups. Resistance band exercises include bicep curls, shoulder presses, and leg extensions.

Incorporating a variety of strength training exercises into your fitness routine is essential for achieving optimal results. Remember to start with proper warm-up and cool-down exercises and consult a fitness professional if you are new to strength training. Stay committed, challenge yourself, and enjoy the benefits of improved strength, endurance, and overall fitness in your journey towards a healthier and fitter life.

Proper Technique and Form

When it comes to physical fitness and exercise, one of the most crucial aspects to consider is proper technique and form. Whether you are a beginner or a seasoned fitness enthusiast, understanding and implementing correct form is essential for maximizing results and preventing injuries. In this subchapter, we will delve into the importance of proper technique and form in various exercises, ensuring that you can achieve your fitness goals safely and effectively.

Proper technique and form are the foundations of any successful exercise routine. Whether you are lifting weights, performing cardiovascular exercises, or engaging in flexibility training, it is essential to learn the correct form from the start. By doing so, you not only optimize the efficiency of your workouts but also minimize the risk of strains, sprains, and other injuries.

For weightlifting exercises, proper technique is paramount. It involves maintaining the correct posture, engaging the appropriate muscles, and executing each movement with control. By learning the correct form, you will engage the targeted muscles more effectively, promoting muscle growth and strength development. Additionally, maintaining proper posture ensures that your joints are properly aligned, reducing the risk of joint pain and injury.

Cardiovascular exercises, such as running, cycling, or swimming, also require proper form to reap maximum benefits. By maintaining proper posture and alignment during these activities, you can enhance your endurance, increase your calorie burn, and reduce the risk of developing overuse injuries. Understanding the proper breathing techniques during cardiovascular exercises is also crucial for improving performance and preventing fatigue.

Flexibility training, which includes activities like yoga or Pilates, relies heavily on proper technique and form to increase flexibility, range of motion, and prevent injuries. By focusing on alignment and form during these exercises, you can target specific muscle groups and improve your overall flexibility. Additionally, proper form ensures that you are engaging the right muscles during each stretch, resulting in a more effective and safe practice.

In conclusion, proper technique and form are fundamental to achieving your fitness goals while maintaining a healthy lifestyle. Whether you are lifting weights, engaging in cardiovascular exercises, or practicing flexibility training, understanding and implementing correct form will optimize your results and minimize the risk of injuries. By prioritizing proper technique, you can ensure that you are making the most out of your workouts and enjoying a long-lasting, fulfilling fitness journey.

Creating a Strength Training Program

Strength training is an essential component of any well-rounded fitness routine. Whether your goal is to improve overall physical fitness, enhance athletic performance, or simply maintain a healthy lifestyle, incorporating strength training exercises into your workout regimen can yield numerous benefits. In this subchapter, we will explore the key elements involved in creating an effective strength training program tailored to meet the needs of adults.

Before embarking on any new exercise regimen, it is crucial to consult with a healthcare professional or certified fitness trainer to ensure that you are physically capable and to receive personalized guidance. Once you have received the green light, it is time to design your strength training program.

The first step in creating a strength training program is to establish your goals. Are you aiming to build muscle mass, increase strength, or improve muscular endurance? Identifying your objectives will allow you to tailor your workouts accordingly. With goals in mind, you can then determine the frequency, duration, and intensity of your strength training sessions.

Next, it is important to select a variety of exercises that target different muscle groups. This can include exercises such as squats, lunges, push-ups, and dumbbell curls, among others. By incorporating a range of movements, you can ensure that you are engaging all major muscle groups and promoting balanced muscular development.

Proper form and technique are fundamental in strength training. To avoid injury and maximize results, it is crucial to learn and maintain correct form for each exercise. Consider working with a fitness professional to learn the proper techniques and ensure that you are performing exercises correctly.

Additionally, it is essential to progressively overload your muscles to continue making gains. This can be achieved by gradually increasing the weight, repetitions, or sets of your exercises over time. However, it is important to listen to your body and avoid overexertion or excessive strain.

In conclusion, creating a strength training program is a vital component of any adult's fitness journey. By establishing clear goals, selecting appropriate exercises, maintaining proper form, and gradually increasing the intensity, you can experience the numerous benefits of strength training, such as improved physical fitness, enhanced athletic performance, and overall health and well-being. Remember to consult with a professional and listen to your body throughout the process to ensure a safe and effective training program.

Chapter 6: Flexibility and Mobility Exercises

Importance of Flexibility and Mobility in Adulthood

As we age, our bodies undergo numerous changes that can impact our overall physical fitness and health. In order to maintain a healthy and active lifestyle, it is essential to prioritize flexibility and mobility in our daily routines. This subchapter aims to highlight the significance of incorporating flexibility and mobility exercises into adulthood, focusing on the niches of physical fitness and exercise, nutrition and healthy eating, and weight loss and a healthy lifestyle.

Physical Fitness and Exercise:

Flexibility and mobility exercises play a crucial role in enhancing physical fitness and exercise routines for adults. Regular stretching and mobility exercises help to improve joint range of motion, prevent injuries, and promote better posture and balance. Incorporating activities such as yoga, Pilates, and tai chi can help maintain flexibility, increase muscle strength, and reduce the risk of age-related conditions like arthritis and osteoporosis. By dedicating time to stretching and mobility exercises, adults can enjoy increased energy levels, improved athletic performance, and a greater sense of overall well-being.

Nutrition and Healthy Eating:

Flexibility and mobility exercises should be complemented by a balanced and nutritious diet. Adequate intake of vitamins and minerals, particularly calcium and vitamin D, is crucial for maintaining bone health and preventing age-related disorders. By consuming a well-balanced diet consisting of fruits, vegetables, lean proteins, whole grains, and healthy fats, adults can support their flexibility and mobility goals. Additionally, staying hydrated is vital for joint lubrication and overall bodily functions. Proper nutrition and hydration can enhance the effectiveness of flexibility and mobility exercises, ensuring optimal results for adults.

Weight Loss and Healthy Lifestyle:

Flexibility and mobility exercises contribute to weight loss and a healthy lifestyle in several ways. Regular physical activity, including stretching and mobility exercises, increases calorie burn, helping to create a calorie deficit necessary for weight loss. Moreover, by improving flexibility and mobility, adults can engage in more diverse exercise routines, which can enhance weight loss efforts. Additionally, incorporating stretching and mobility exercises into daily routines can alleviate stress, improve sleep quality, and enhance overall mental well-being, all of which are essential for maintaining a healthy lifestyle.

Conclusion:

In conclusion, flexibility and mobility exercises are crucial for maintaining physical fitness, supporting proper nutrition, and promoting weight loss and a healthy lifestyle in adulthood. By incorporating regular stretching and mobility exercises into our routines, adults can enjoy enhanced joint health, increased energy levels, improved physical performance, and reduced risk of age-related conditions. Furthermore, when combined with a balanced diet and overall healthy lifestyle habits, flexibility and mobility exercises can lead to a happier, healthier, and more fulfilling adulthood.

Stretching Exercises for Improved Flexibility

Introduction:
Flexibility is an essential component of physical fitness that often gets overlooked. Many adults focus solely on cardiovascular exercises or strength training, neglecting the importance of maintaining and improving their flexibility. However, incorporating stretching exercises into your fitness routine can offer numerous benefits, such as increased range of motion, improved posture, reduced muscle tension, and enhanced athletic performance. In this subchapter, we will explore various stretching exercises that adults can incorporate into their daily routines to improve flexibility and overall physical fitness.

1. Dynamic Stretching:
Dynamic stretching involves moving parts of your body through a full range of motion. It is particularly beneficial for warming up the muscles before a workout. Exercises such as arm circles, leg swings, and torso twists can help increase blood flow, warm up the muscles, and prepare your body for more intense activities.

2. Static Stretching:
Static stretching involves holding a stretch for an extended period, typically around 30 seconds to one minute. This type of stretching is best performed after your workout or any physical activity when the muscles are warm. Static stretches help improve muscle flexibility and can include exercises like hamstring stretches, calf stretches, and shoulder stretches.

3. Yoga and Pilates:
Yoga and Pilates are popular practices known for their emphasis on flexibility, strength, and mindfulness. These disciplines combine stretching exercises with deep breathing and bodyweight resistance movements. Incorporating yoga or Pilates into your fitness routine can help increase overall flexibility while also promoting relaxation and mental well-being.

4. Foam Rolling:
Foam rolling, also known as self-myofascial release, involves using a foam roller to apply pressure to specific areas of the body. This technique helps release muscle knots and tension, promoting better flexibility and muscle recovery. Foam rolling can be particularly beneficial for adults who experience muscle tightness due to prolonged sitting or physical activities.

Conclusion:
Improving flexibility through stretching exercises is crucial for adults looking to enhance physical fitness, maintain joint health, and prevent injuries. Whether you choose dynamic or static stretching, incorporate yoga or Pilates into your routine, or use foam rolling techniques, regular stretching exercises can lead to improved flexibility and overall well-being. Remember to consult with a fitness professional or healthcare provider before starting any new exercise program, especially if you have any pre-existing medical conditions. By dedicating a few minutes each day to stretching, you can unlock the benefits of improved flexibility and enjoy a healthier, more active lifestyle.

Incorporating Mobility Exercises in Your Routine

When it comes to achieving optimal physical fitness and maintaining a healthy lifestyle, exercise is paramount. However, many adults overlook the importance of incorporating mobility exercises into their routine. Mobility exercises focus on improving joint function, flexibility, and range of motion, which are critical for overall well-being.

Why are mobility exercises important? As we age, our joints naturally become stiffer, and our muscles tend to tighten. This can lead to reduced mobility, increased risk of injury, and even chronic pain. By incorporating mobility exercises into your routine, you can counteract these effects and maintain your physical independence.

One of the most significant benefits of mobility exercises is their ability to improve joint health. Regular mobility exercises increase the synovial fluid's production, which lubricates the joints, reducing friction and enhancing their function. By keeping your joints healthy, you can prevent conditions like osteoarthritis and maintain your active lifestyle.

Flexibility and range of motion are also crucial for overall physical fitness. By performing mobility exercises, you can improve your flexibility, allowing you to move more freely and efficiently during other exercises and daily activities. These exercises will also help you maintain a good posture, reducing the risk of back pain and other musculoskeletal issues.

Incorporating mobility exercises into your routine doesn't have to be complicated or time-consuming. Simple exercises like neck rotations, shoulder rolls, and ankle circles can be done anywhere, anytime. You can also try yoga or Pilates classes, which focus on enhancing flexibility and joint mobility.

It's important to note that mobility exercises should complement your existing workout routine. By incorporating them as a warm-up or cool-down activity, you can prepare your body for more intense exercises and reduce the risk of injury.

In addition to mobility exercises, maintaining a balanced diet is essential for overall health and well-being. Proper nutrition provides the necessary nutrients for joint health and muscle repair, ensuring that your body functions optimally. Focus on consuming a variety of fruits, vegetables, lean proteins, and whole grains to support your fitness goals.

In conclusion, incorporating mobility exercises into your routine is crucial for maintaining physical fitness, preventing injury, and promoting a healthy lifestyle. By improving joint health, flexibility, and range of motion, you can enhance your overall well-being and enjoy a more active and pain-free life. Remember to consult with a healthcare professional or a certified fitness trainer before starting any new exercise program.

Chapter 7: Nutrition and Healthy Eating Habits

Understanding Macronutrients and Micronutrients

In order to achieve optimal physical fitness and maintain a healthy lifestyle, it is essential to understand the importance of macronutrients and micronutrients. These two categories of nutrients play a crucial role in providing the body with the necessary fuel and building blocks for overall health and wellbeing.

Macronutrients are the nutrients that the body needs in large quantities to function properly. They include carbohydrates, proteins, and fats. Carbohydrates are the body's main source of energy and are found in foods such as grains, fruits, and vegetables. Proteins are essential for building and repairing tissues, as well as supporting the immune system. Good sources of protein include lean meats, fish, dairy products, and legumes. Fats, although often demonized, are actually vital for many bodily functions and provide a concentrated source of energy. Healthy fats can be found in foods like avocados, nuts, and olive oil.

On the other hand, micronutrients are nutrients that the body requires in smaller amounts but are equally important for overall health. These include vitamins and minerals. Vitamins are organic compounds that are necessary for various physiological functions, such as cell growth, immune system support, and energy production. They can be obtained from a balanced diet that includes a variety of fruits, vegetables, and whole grains. Minerals, on the other hand, are inorganic compounds that are essential for maintaining proper bodily functions, including bone health, nerve function, and fluid balance. Minerals can be found in foods like leafy greens, nuts, seeds, and dairy products.

Understanding the role of macronutrients and micronutrients is essential for achieving and maintaining a healthy weight. By consuming the right balance of carbohydrates, proteins, and fats, individuals can fuel their bodies for physical activity while also supporting muscle growth and repair. Additionally, ensuring an adequate intake of vitamins and minerals is crucial for overall health and preventing deficiencies that can lead to a range of health issues.

In conclusion, a balanced understanding of macronutrients and micronutrients is essential for individuals seeking to improve their physical fitness and maintain a healthy lifestyle. By incorporating a variety of nutrient-dense foods into their diet, individuals can provide their bodies with the necessary fuel and building blocks for optimal health and wellbeing. So, whether you are looking to lose weight, improve your fitness level, or simply live a healthier life, paying attention to macronutrients and micronutrients is key.

The Role of Protein, Carbohydrates, and Fats in a Balanced Diet

In our quest for physical fitness and a healthy lifestyle, it is crucial to understand the role of protein, carbohydrates, and fats in maintaining a balanced diet. These macronutrients play a vital role in providing energy, supporting muscle growth and repair, and ensuring overall well-being. In this subchapter, we will delve into the importance of these nutrients and how to incorporate them into our daily diet.

Protein is often referred to as the building block of life, and rightfully so. It is essential for repairing and building tissues, including muscles, skin, and organs. It also plays a crucial role in the production of enzymes and hormones, aiding in various bodily functions. Including lean sources of protein, such as chicken, turkey, fish, tofu, and legumes, in our diet is essential. These foods not only provide essential amino acids but also help in maintaining satiety and promoting weight loss.

Carbohydrates are the primary source of energy for our bodies. They are broken down into glucose, which fuels our cells and powers our physical activities. However, not all carbohydrates are created equal. Opting for complex carbohydrates, such as whole grains, vegetables, and fruits, is recommended. These sources provide essential vitamins, minerals, and fiber, ensuring a steady release of energy and preventing blood sugar spikes.

Contrary to popular belief, fats are an essential part of a healthy diet. They provide energy, aid in nutrient absorption, and protect organs. However, it is important to choose healthy fats, such as those found in avocados, nuts, seeds, and olive oil, over saturated and trans fats. Healthy fats promote heart health, reduce inflammation, and support brain function.

Balancing these macronutrients is crucial for weight loss and healthy living. Opting for a diet that includes a combination of lean protein, complex carbohydrates, and healthy fats helps to control cravings, maintain energy levels, and achieve and sustain a healthy weight. It is important to note that the proportion of these macronutrients may vary depending on individual goals, activity levels, and overall health.

In conclusion, protein, carbohydrates, and fats are all essential components of a well-rounded and balanced diet. Understanding the role of these macronutrients and incorporating them in appropriate proportions can significantly impact our physical fitness, nutrition, and overall well-being. By making informed choices and embracing a balanced approach to nutrition, we can achieve our fitness goals and lead a healthier lifestyle.

Portion Control and Mindful Eating

In our fast-paced and convenience-driven world, it's easy to lose sight of the importance of portion control and mindful eating. However, these two practices are crucial when it comes to achieving and maintaining a healthy lifestyle. Whether your goal is physical fitness, nutrition, weight loss, or all of the above, mastering portion control and mindful eating will undoubtedly contribute to your success.

Portion control is the practice of being mindful of the amount of food you consume in one sitting. It involves understanding serving sizes and listening to your body's hunger and fullness cues. Many of us are guilty of mindlessly eating oversized portions, which can lead to weight gain and other health issues. By practicing portion control, you can ensure that you are consuming the right amount of nutrients for your body's needs.

Mindful eating, on the other hand, goes beyond portion control. It is about being fully present and engaged during your meals, paying attention to the flavors, textures, and sensations of each bite. Mindful eating encourages you to listen to your body's hunger and fullness signals, as well as to recognize and address emotional or stress-related eating triggers. By practicing mindful eating, you can foster a healthier relationship with food, reduce overeating, and make more conscious choices about what and how you eat.

To incorporate portion control and mindful eating into your daily routine, start by becoming aware of your current eating habits. Take note of the portion sizes you typically consume and whether you tend to eat quickly or mindlessly. Consider using smaller plates and bowls to help control portion sizes, and take the time to savor each bite by chewing slowly and putting your utensils down between bites.

Additionally, try to eliminate distractions during mealtime, such as watching TV or scrolling through your phone. Instead, focus on the food in front of you and the experience of eating. Pay attention to your body's hunger and fullness signals, and stop eating when you feel satisfied, rather than overly full.

Remember, portion control and mindful eating are lifelong practices that require patience and consistency. It's not about deprivation or strict rules; rather, it's about finding balance and enjoying food in a way that nourishes your body and mind. By incorporating these practices into your daily routine, you can optimize your physical fitness, improve your nutrition, and achieve your weight loss goals, all while fostering a healthier and more mindful approach to eating.

Strategies for Healthy Meal Planning and Preparation

In our fast-paced modern lives, it can be challenging to prioritize our health and make wise choices when it comes to our meals. However, with proper planning and preparation, we can easily incorporate healthy eating habits into our daily routines. This subchapter aims to provide you with strategies for effective meal planning and preparation, ensuring that you maintain a nutritious diet while pursuing your fitness goals.

1. Set Realistic Goals: Begin by setting realistic goals for your meal planning and preparation. Consider your dietary requirements, fitness objectives, and personal preferences. This will help you focus on creating a well-balanced and tailored meal plan that suits your needs.

2. Plan Ahead: Dedicate some time each week to plan your meals in advance. This will save you time, reduce stress, and prevent impulsive food choices. Decide on the number of meals you want to prepare and create a shopping list accordingly.

3. Include a Variety of Nutrient-Dense Foods: Aim to incorporate a variety of nutrient-dense foods into your meals. Include a good balance of lean proteins, whole grains, fruits, vegetables, and healthy fats. Experiment with different recipes and flavors to keep your meals interesting.

4. Portion Control: Be mindful of portion sizes to avoid overeating. Use smaller plates and bowls to help control portion sizes visually. Include adequate servings of protein, carbohydrates, and healthy fats to ensure you meet your nutritional requirements.

5. Batch Cooking and Meal Prep: Consider batch cooking and meal prepping on weekends or days off. Cook larger portions of meals that can be divided into individual servings and stored for later use. This will save you time during busy weekdays and help you make healthier choices.

6. Make Use of Technology: Utilize meal planning and tracking apps to simplify the process. These apps offer recipe suggestions, grocery lists, and even calorie tracking features, making it easier to manage your meals and monitor your progress.

7. Mindful Eating: Practice mindful eating by savoring each bite and paying attention to your body's hunger and fullness cues. Avoid distractions while eating, such as watching TV or using electronic devices. This will help you appreciate your meals and prevent overeating.

By implementing these strategies, you can take control of your meal planning and preparation, leading to a healthier and more balanced lifestyle. Remember, it's not only about what you eat but also how you prepare and consume your meals that contribute to your overall well-being. Start incorporating these habits into your routine, and you will be well on your way to achieving your fitness and nutrition goals.

Chapter 8: Weight Loss Strategies for Adults

Understanding Weight Loss Principles and Myths

In the pursuit of a healthy lifestyle, weight loss is often a primary goal for many adults. However, the path to shedding those extra pounds is often paved with misconceptions and myths. In this subchapter, we will delve into the principles of weight loss, debunk prevalent myths, and provide you with the knowledge to achieve your goals effectively.

Firstly, it is crucial to understand that weight loss is a complex process that involves both the body and the mind. Sustainable weight loss is not about crash diets or overnight miracles; it is a gradual and holistic transformation. It requires a balance between physical fitness, nutrition, and healthy eating habits.

One common misconception is that weight loss is solely about caloric restriction. While creating a calorie deficit is essential for shedding pounds, it is equally important to focus on the quality of the calories consumed. Opting for nutrient-dense foods such as fruits, vegetables, lean proteins, and whole grains should be the foundation of any weight loss plan.

Another myth often perpetuated is that all calories are created equal. In reality, the body processes different types of calories differently. For instance, consuming 100 calories from an apple versus 100 calories from a sugary beverage will have vastly different impacts on your body. Understanding the importance of macronutrients, such as carbohydrates, proteins, and fats, is crucial in developing a balanced and effective weight loss strategy.

Furthermore, exercise plays a significant role in weight loss. Implementing a regular exercise routine not only burns calories but also improves overall health and well-being. Combining cardiovascular exercises, strength training, and flexibility exercises can help boost metabolism, build lean muscle mass, and accelerate weight loss.

While weight loss myths may promise quick results, they often lead to disappointment and frustration. Understanding the principles of weight loss and adopting a healthy lifestyle is the key to achieving sustainable and long-lasting results. By focusing on a balanced diet, regular exercise, and a positive mindset, you can embark on a journey towards a healthier, fitter, and more confident you.

In conclusion, understanding weight loss principles and dispelling the myths surrounding it is vital for anyone striving to achieve a healthy lifestyle. By embracing the principles of nutrition, exercise, and a positive mindset, you can embark on a transformative journey towards weight loss success. Remember, sustainable weight loss is not a sprint but a marathon, and with the right knowledge and dedication, you can achieve your goals and thrive in your pursuit of physical fitness and overall well-being.

Creating a Calorie Deficit for Weight Loss

When it comes to achieving weight loss goals, creating a calorie deficit is a fundamental concept that should not be overlooked. In this subchapter, we will explore the importance of a calorie deficit and how it can be achieved to promote successful weight loss.

To put it simply, a calorie deficit occurs when you consume fewer calories than your body needs to maintain its current weight. This deficit forces your body to tap into its energy reserves, resulting in weight loss. While this concept may seem straightforward, it is important to approach it with a balanced and sustainable mindset.

First and foremost, it is crucial to understand your body's daily caloric needs. This can be determined by factors such as your age, weight, height, and activity level. Consulting with a registered dietitian or utilizing online calculators can provide you with a rough estimate of your daily caloric needs. Once you have this number, you can begin creating a calorie deficit.

There are two primary ways to create a calorie deficit: through diet and exercise. When it comes to your diet, focus on making healthier food choices and reducing portion sizes. Incorporate more whole foods such as fruits, vegetables, lean proteins, and whole grains into your meals. These foods are not only lower in calories, but they also provide essential nutrients that support overall health.

In addition to modifying your diet, exercise plays a crucial role in creating a calorie deficit. Engaging in regular physical activity not only burns calories but also boosts your metabolism, making weight loss more sustainable. Find activities that you enjoy, whether it's jogging, swimming, dancing, or attending fitness classes. Aim for at least 150 minutes of moderate-intensity exercise or 75 minutes of vigorous-intensity exercise per week.

Remember, creating a calorie deficit should be approached with a balanced mindset. Drastically cutting calories or overexerting yourself with excessive exercise can be detrimental to your health and hinder your weight loss progress. Aim for a gradual and realistic approach that allows for long-term success.

In conclusion, creating a calorie deficit is a key component of successful weight loss. By understanding your daily caloric needs, making healthier food choices, and engaging in regular physical activity, you can achieve a sustainable calorie deficit and reach your weight loss goals. Always prioritize your overall health and well-being throughout this journey.

Incorporating Physical Activity for Weight Loss

Physical activity is an essential component of any weight loss journey. It not only helps you shed those extra pounds but also improves your overall health and well-being. In this subchapter, we will explore how you can incorporate physical activity into your daily routine to achieve your weight loss goals.

When it comes to weight loss, the first thing to remember is that there is no one-size-fits-all approach. Every individual is unique, and what works for one person may not work for another. However, there are some universal principles that can guide you in incorporating physical activity into your weight loss plan.

The key to successful weight loss is finding activities that you enjoy and that fit into your lifestyle. This could be anything from walking or running to dancing, swimming, or cycling. The options are endless, so choose activities that you find enjoyable and that align with your interests. By doing so, you are more likely to stick with them in the long run.

It is recommended that adults engage in at least 150 minutes of moderate-intensity aerobic activity or 75 minutes of vigorous-intensity aerobic activity per week. This can be broken down into smaller sessions throughout the week to make it more manageable. Additionally, incorporating strength training exercises at least two days a week can help build lean muscle mass, boost your metabolism, and aid in weight loss.

To make physical activity a habit, try to schedule it into your daily routine. Treat it as an appointment with yourself that you cannot miss. Block off time in your calendar, set reminders, and make it a priority. You can also enlist the support of a workout buddy or join a fitness class or group to stay motivated and accountable.

Remember that physical activity alone is not enough for weight loss. It should be complemented by a balanced and nutritious diet. Focus on consuming whole, unprocessed foods, and aim to create a calorie deficit by reducing portion sizes and choosing healthier alternatives. Consulting a nutritionist or registered dietitian can provide valuable guidance in designing a meal plan that supports your weight loss goals.

Incorporating physical activity for weight loss requires commitment, consistency, and patience. It is a journey that may have its ups and downs, but with determination and the right mindset, you can achieve your desired results. So lace up your sneakers, find an activity that brings you joy, and start moving towards a healthier, fitter, and more vibrant life.

Tips for Sustainable Weight Loss and Maintenance

Introduction:
Losing weight is often a challenging journey, but it becomes even more crucial to sustain it in the long term. This subchapter aims to provide you with valuable tips for sustainable weight loss and maintenance. By following these guidelines, you will not only achieve your weight loss goals but also develop a healthy lifestyle for a lifetime.

1. Set Realistic Goals:
When embarking on a weight loss journey, it is essential to set realistic and achievable goals. Aim for a gradual weight loss of 1-2 pounds per week. This approach ensures that you are losing fat rather than muscle and allows your body to adjust to the changes gradually.

2. Prioritize Physical Activity:
Regular exercise plays a vital role in weight loss and maintenance. Engage in a combination of cardiovascular exercises and strength training to burn calories and build lean muscle mass. Find activities you enjoy, such as jogging, swimming, or cycling, and aim for at least 150 minutes of moderate-intensity exercise per week.

3. Adopt a Balanced Diet:
Nutrition is key to sustainable weight loss. Focus on consuming a balanced diet that includes whole grains, lean proteins, fruits, vegetables, and healthy fats. Avoid fad diets that promise quick results but are difficult to maintain in the long run. Instead, aim for a lifestyle change by making healthier food choices.

4. Practice Portion Control:
Controlling portion sizes is crucial for weight loss and maintenance. Use smaller plates and bowls to control the amount of food you eat. Pay attention to your body's hunger and fullness cues, and avoid eating until you are overly stuffed. Be mindful of mindless snacking, as it can contribute to weight gain.

5. Stay Hydrated:

Water is essential for overall health and weight management. Ensure you drink an adequate amount of water throughout the day to stay hydrated and curb unnecessary snacking. Replace sugary beverages with water or herbal teas to reduce calorie intake.

6. Get Adequate Sleep:

Sleep plays a crucial role in maintaining a healthy weight. Lack of sleep can disrupt hormones that regulate appetite, leading to increased cravings and overeating. Aim for 7-9 hours of quality sleep each night to support your weight loss efforts.

7. Seek Support and Accountability:

Having a support system can greatly contribute to sustainable weight loss. Join a weight loss group, enlist a workout buddy, or seek professional help from a registered dietitian or personal trainer. Their guidance and encouragement will help you stay motivated and on track.

Conclusion:

Sustainable weight loss and maintenance require a holistic approach that combines physical activity, a balanced diet, and healthy lifestyle habits. By setting realistic goals, prioritizing exercise, adopting a balanced diet, controlling portions, staying hydrated, getting enough sleep, and seeking support, you will be on your way to achieving and maintaining a healthy weight for life. Remember, it's not just about reaching a number on the scale; it's about establishing lifelong habits that promote overall well-being.

Chapter 9: Maintaining a Healthy Lifestyle

Incorporating Exercise and Healthy Eating into Your Daily Routine

Maintaining a healthy lifestyle requires a combination of regular exercise and a balanced diet. By incorporating exercise and healthy eating into your daily routine, you can achieve optimal physical fitness, improve nutrition habits, and even shed unwanted pounds. This subchapter will provide you with practical tips and strategies to help you make these essential changes and lead a healthier, more fulfilling life.

Regular exercise is key to overall physical fitness. Adults should aim for at least 150 minutes of moderate-intensity aerobic activity or 75 minutes of vigorous-intensity aerobic activity each week. This can include activities such as brisk walking, jogging, cycling, swimming, or group fitness classes. By scheduling exercise into your daily routine, you can improve cardiovascular health, strengthen muscles, and boost your mood.

To make exercise a habit, find activities you enjoy and vary your routine to keep things interesting. Consider incorporating strength training exercises to build muscle mass and increase metabolism. Additionally, make it a priority to engage in regular stretching and flexibility exercises to improve joint mobility and prevent injuries.

While exercise is crucial, it is equally important to fuel your body with proper nutrition. A healthy eating plan should include a variety of fruits, vegetables, whole grains, lean proteins, and healthy fats. Aim to consume nutrient-dense foods that are low in added sugars, sodium, and unhealthy fats.

To develop healthy eating habits, plan your meals and snacks in advance. Prepare nutritious meals at home using fresh ingredients, and limit your intake of processed foods and takeout meals. Be mindful of portion sizes and practice mindful eating to savor the flavors and listen to your body's hunger and fullness cues.

Incorporating exercise and healthy eating into your daily routine will not only improve your physical fitness but also aid in weight loss. By burning calories through exercise and consuming a balanced diet, you can create a calorie deficit that promotes gradual and sustainable weight loss. Remember, consistency is key, so make these changes a long-term commitment rather than a short-lived diet or exercise program.

In conclusion, this subchapter highlights the importance of incorporating exercise and healthy eating into your daily routine. By prioritizing physical fitness, improving nutrition habits, and maintaining a healthy weight, you can enjoy a happier, more energized, and fulfilling life. Take the first step towards a healthier lifestyle today by implementing these strategies and reaping the long-term benefits they offer.

Strategies for Overcoming Plateaus and Staying Motivated

Plateaus are a common occurrence in any fitness journey. They can be frustrating and demotivating, but they are not insurmountable. In this subchapter, we will explore effective strategies to overcome plateaus and stay motivated on your path to physical fitness and a healthy lifestyle.

1. Mix Up Your Exercise Routine: One of the main reasons for plateaus is your body getting used to a particular exercise routine. To break through, try incorporating different types of exercises, such as cardio, strength training, and flexibility exercises. This not only challenges your body but also prevents boredom.

2. Set Realistic Goals: Plateaus often occur when we have unrealistic expectations. Instead of focusing solely on weight loss or achieving a specific body shape, set goals that include overall health improvement, increased stamina, or achieving a certain level of flexibility. Celebrate these milestones to keep yourself motivated.

3. Track Your Progress: Keep a record of your workouts, measurements, and any changes you notice in your body. This will help you see the progress you've made, even when it may not be immediately visible. Seeing your accomplishments can reignite your motivation and help you push through plateaus.

4. Find an Accountability Partner: Having someone to hold you accountable can make a world of difference. Find a workout buddy or join a fitness group where you can support and motivate each other. Share your goals, challenges, and achievements, and lean on each other during the tough times.

5. Reward Yourself: Treat yourself when you reach certain milestones. It could be buying new workout gear, going for a spa day, or indulging in a favorite healthy meal. These rewards act as positive reinforcement and give you something to strive for.

6. Get Professional Guidance: Consider working with a personal trainer or a nutritionist to help you navigate through plateaus. They can provide expert advice, tailor a workout or nutrition plan to your specific needs, and provide the motivation and support you need to break through.

Remember, plateaus are a normal part of the fitness journey. The key is to stay committed and motivated. By implementing these strategies, you can overcome plateaus, achieve your fitness goals, and live a healthy and fulfilling life. Keep pushing yourself, and the results will follow.

Stress Management and its Impact on Physical Fitness

In today's fast-paced world, stress has become an inevitable part of our lives. Juggling work, family, and personal commitments can leave us feeling overwhelmed and drained. However, understanding the importance of stress management and its impact on physical fitness is crucial for leading a healthy and balanced lifestyle.

Stress, if left unmanaged, can take a toll on our physical well-being. It triggers the release of cortisol, a hormone that, when elevated for prolonged periods, can lead to weight gain, high blood pressure, and weakened immune function. This can be detrimental to our overall health and hinder our fitness goals.

One of the most effective ways to manage stress and improve physical fitness is through regular exercise. Engaging in physical activity releases endorphins, also known as the "feel-good" hormones, which help reduce stress and improve mood. Whether it's a brisk walk, a yoga session, or a high-intensity workout, finding an exercise routine that suits your preferences can significantly reduce stress levels and enhance overall well-being.

In addition to exercise, nutrition plays a vital role in stress management. A well-balanced diet rich in fruits, vegetables, lean proteins, and whole grains provides the necessary nutrients to combat stress. Avoiding processed foods, caffeine, and excessive sugar can help stabilize blood sugar levels and prevent energy crashes, which often exacerbate stress. Incorporating stress-busting foods such as dark chocolate, nuts, and green leafy vegetables can also provide a natural boost to your mood and overall health.

Moreover, adopting a healthy lifestyle and maintaining a healthy weight can positively impact stress levels. Excess weight puts additional strain on the body, leading to increased stress. By focusing on weight loss and healthy living, individuals can reduce their risk of chronic conditions associated with stress, such as heart disease and diabetes.

In conclusion, stress management is essential for maintaining physical fitness and overall well-being. By incorporating regular exercise, a nutritious diet, and adopting a healthy lifestyle, adults can effectively manage stress levels and improve their physical fitness. Understanding the impact of stress on our bodies is the first step towards leading a balanced and fulfilling life. Remember, taking care of yourself is not a luxury but a necessity, and stress management plays a crucial role in achieving optimal physical fitness and overall health.

Creating a Supportive Environment for Your Healthy Lifestyle

In our quest for a healthier lifestyle, it's crucial to understand that our environment plays a significant role in our success. To truly thrive in our journey towards physical fitness and overall well-being, we need to create a supportive environment that nurtures our goals and aspirations. This subchapter explores practical strategies to transform your surroundings into a sanctuary that fosters a healthy lifestyle.

First and foremost, let's focus on physical fitness and exercise. Ensure you have a designated workout space at home, whether it's a spare room or a corner of your living room. Remove any clutter or distractions that may hinder your workout sessions. Consider investing in equipment that aligns with your fitness goals, such as dumbbells, resistance bands, or a yoga mat. By creating a dedicated workout space, you are more likely to prioritize exercise and make it a regular part of your routine.

Next, let's delve into the realm of nutrition and healthy eating. The key here is to set yourself up for success by organizing your kitchen and pantry. Rid your shelves of unhealthy temptations and replace them with nutritious options. Stock up on fresh fruits, vegetables, whole grains, and lean proteins. Keep your kitchen well-stocked with essential cooking tools and gadgets. This will make meal preparation easier and more enjoyable, encouraging you to cook nutritious meals at home rather than relying on fast food or processed options.

Weight loss and adopting a healthy lifestyle can be challenging, but with the right environment, you can make it easier on yourself. Surround yourself with like-minded individuals who share your goals and values. Join fitness classes, clubs, or online communities where you can connect with others on a similar journey. Having a support system will provide you with motivation, accountability, and a sense of camaraderie.

Lastly, it's essential to make your home a sanctuary of relaxation and stress relief. Create a calming environment by incorporating elements such as soft lighting, soothing colors, and comfortable furniture. Dedicate a space for mindfulness activities like meditation or yoga. Engaging in these practices regularly will help reduce stress levels and promote overall well-being.

Remember, creating a supportive environment is a continuous process. Regularly assess your surroundings and make adjustments as needed. By taking the time to cultivate an environment that supports your healthy lifestyle, you are setting yourself up for long-term success and a fulfilling journey towards physical fitness and overall wellness.

Chapter 10: Common Challenges and Solutions for Adults

Overcoming Time Constraints and Busy Schedules

In today's fast-paced world, it can be challenging for adults to find time for physical fitness and exercise. With demanding work schedules, family responsibilities, and numerous other obligations, it's no wonder that many adults struggle to prioritize their health and well-being. However, with the right mindset and strategies, it is possible to overcome time constraints and incorporate fitness into even the busiest of schedules.

First and foremost, it's essential to recognize the importance of physical fitness and exercise for overall health. Regular exercise not only helps maintain a healthy weight but also reduces the risk of chronic diseases, boosts mood, and improves energy levels. By understanding the significant benefits, adults can find the motivation to make fitness a priority in their lives.

One effective strategy for overcoming time constraints is to schedule workouts like any other important appointment. By blocking off specific times in your calendar for exercise, you are more likely to follow through and make it a habit. Whether it's waking up early for a morning jog, utilizing your lunch break for a quick workout, or dedicating time in the evenings, finding a consistent routine that suits your schedule is key.

Moreover, it's crucial to make the most of the time available. High-intensity interval training (HIIT) workouts, for example, offer a quick and intense burst of exercise that can be completed in as little as 15 minutes. These workouts combine short bursts of intense activity with brief recovery periods, maximizing calorie burn and cardiovascular benefits in a short amount of time.

Additionally, incorporating physical activity into daily routines can help overcome time constraints. Instead of taking the elevator, opt for the stairs. Park your car further away from your destination and walk the extra distance. Take breaks throughout the workday to stretch and move around. These small changes may seem insignificant, but they add up and contribute to overall fitness and well-being.

Lastly, it's essential to remember that nutrition plays a significant role in maintaining a healthy lifestyle. Planning and preparing meals in advance can help save time and ensure you have nutritious options readily available. Batch cooking on weekends, utilizing slow cookers, and creating meal plans can make healthy eating more manageable, even with a busy schedule.

In conclusion, while time constraints and busy schedules can be challenging, it is possible for adults to prioritize physical fitness and exercise. By recognizing the importance of fitness, scheduling workouts, making the most of available time, and incorporating physical activity into daily routines, adults can overcome obstacles and achieve a healthy and active lifestyle. Remember, small steps and consistent effort can lead to significant long-term results.

Dealing with Injuries and Physical Limitations

In our journey towards physical fitness and overall well-being, it is important to acknowledge that injuries and physical limitations can sometimes hinder our progress. Whether it's a sprained ankle, a chronic condition, or a past injury, these challenges can make it difficult to maintain our exercise routines and reach our fitness goals. However, with the right knowledge and mindset, we can still lead a healthy and active lifestyle.

First and foremost, it is crucial to listen to your body. If you experience pain or discomfort during exercise, it's essential to stop and assess the situation. Pushing through the pain can exacerbate the injury and lead to further setbacks. Instead, take the time to rest and allow your body to heal. Consult with a healthcare professional, such as a physical therapist or a sports medicine specialist, who can provide guidance on how to manage your injury or limitation.

While you may not be able to engage in your usual exercise routine, it doesn't mean you have to give up physical activity altogether. There are various low-impact exercises and alternative workout options that can help you stay active without putting unnecessary strain on your injury. For example, if you have a knee injury, swimming or cycling can provide cardiovascular benefits without placing excessive stress on your joints.

In addition to modifying your exercise routine, nutrition plays a vital role in supporting your body's healing process. Focus on consuming a well-balanced diet rich in nutrients that aid in recovery, such as lean proteins, fruits, vegetables, and whole grains. Consider incorporating foods with anti-inflammatory properties, like turmeric and fatty fish, to reduce inflammation and promote healing.

It's also crucial to be patient and kind to yourself during this time. Remember that setbacks are a part of the journey, and it's essential to give yourself grace. Celebrate the small victories and focus on what you can do rather than what you can't. Seek support from friends, family, or online communities that share similar experiences to stay motivated and inspired.

Ultimately, dealing with injuries and physical limitations is a challenge that many of us face at some point in our lives. By adapting our approach, seeking professional guidance, and staying committed to our overall well-being, we can overcome these obstacles and continue on our path towards a fit and healthy life. Remember, it's not about perfection; it's about progress.

Addressing Mental and Emotional Barriers to Exercise

In our quest for physical fitness and a healthy lifestyle, we often focus solely on the physical aspects such as exercise routines and nutrition plans. However, we tend to overlook the significant impact that mental and emotional barriers can have on our ability to maintain a consistent exercise regimen. In this subchapter, we will explore the various mental and emotional barriers that adults may face when trying to adopt a fitness routine and provide practical strategies to overcome them.

One of the most common mental barriers to exercise is a lack of motivation. Many adults struggle to find the drive to start and stick to an exercise program. This lack of motivation may stem from negative self-talk, past failures, or a general feeling of being overwhelmed. To overcome this barrier, it is important to set realistic goals, break them down into smaller, achievable milestones, and celebrate each success along the way. Surrounding yourself with a supportive community, such as workout buddies or joining fitness classes, can also provide the necessary motivation and accountability.

Emotional barriers, such as stress and anxiety, can also hinder our exercise efforts. The demands of daily life, work pressures, and personal challenges can leave us feeling mentally drained and devoid of energy. It is crucial to recognize the connection between physical activity and mental well-being. Engaging in exercise releases endorphins, which are natural mood boosters. Incorporating stress-reducing activities, such as yoga or meditation, into your exercise routine can further alleviate emotional barriers and enhance overall mental health.

Another common mental barrier is the fear of failure or embarrassment. Many adults feel self-conscious about their fitness level or appearance, which prevents them from joining group exercise classes or going to the gym. It is important to remember that everyone starts somewhere, and everyone has their own journey. Embracing a growth mindset and focusing on personal progress rather than comparing oneself to others can help overcome these fears. Starting with low-impact activities, such as walking or swimming, can also build confidence and gradually increase fitness levels.

In conclusion, addressing mental and emotional barriers is crucial for adults striving for physical fitness and a healthy lifestyle. By understanding and proactively tackling these barriers, individuals can pave the way for long-term success. Remember, your mental and emotional well-being is just as important as your physical health, and by addressing them, you will be well on your way to achieving a balanced and fulfilling life.

Finding Balance and Long-term Success in Physical Fitness

In today's fast-paced world, finding balance and long-term success in physical fitness can be a challenging endeavor. With work, family, and other commitments, it can be difficult to prioritize our health and well-being. However, by making small changes and adopting a holistic approach, we can achieve our fitness goals while maintaining a balanced and fulfilling lifestyle.

One key aspect of finding balance in physical fitness is incorporating regular exercise into our daily routine. Whether it's going for a jog, attending a yoga class, or hitting the gym, finding an activity that we enjoy is crucial. By making exercise a habit, we can improve our cardiovascular health, build strength, and boost our mood. It's important to remember that consistency is key; even small amounts of exercise done regularly can have a significant impact on our overall fitness.

Another crucial element of long-term success in physical fitness is nutrition and healthy eating. Fueling our bodies with the right nutrients is essential for optimal performance and recovery. A well-balanced diet consisting of lean proteins, whole grains, fruits, and vegetables will provide us with the energy and nutrients we need to reach our fitness goals. It's important to avoid crash diets or extreme restrictions, as they are not sustainable in the long run. Instead, focus on making small, sustainable changes to our eating habits that we can maintain over time.

Weight loss and maintaining a healthy lifestyle go hand in hand with finding balance in physical fitness. While it's natural to desire quick results, it's important to approach weight loss in a healthy and sustainable manner. Crash diets or extreme exercise routines may yield temporary results, but they can be detrimental to our overall well-being. Instead, focus on creating a lifestyle that supports a healthy weight through regular exercise and balanced nutrition.

Finding balance and long-term success in physical fitness is not just about the number on the scale or achieving a specific aesthetic. It's about building a strong foundation of health and well-being that will carry us through all aspects of our lives. By prioritizing our physical fitness, adopting a balanced approach to nutrition, and focusing on long-term sustainability, we can achieve our goals while still enjoying the journey. Remember, it's not just about the destination, but the lifelong commitment to living a healthy and fulfilling life.

Conclusion: Embracing a Fit and Healthy Life as an Adult

In the journey of life, adulthood is a crucial phase where we face numerous challenges, responsibilities, and changes. It is during this time that we must prioritize our physical fitness, nutrition, and overall well-being to lead a fulfilling and healthy life. In this concluding chapter, we will summarize the key takeaways from our book, "Fit for Life: The Ultimate Guide to Physical Fitness and Exercise for Adults," and emphasize the importance of embracing a fit and healthy lifestyle.

Physical fitness and exercise are vital aspects of adult life. Regular exercise not only helps us maintain a healthy weight but also improves our cardiovascular health, strengthens our muscles and bones, and enhances our mental well-being. By incorporating exercise into our daily routine, we can experience increased energy levels, reduced stress, and improved sleep patterns. Whether it's engaging in cardiovascular activities like jogging, swimming, or cycling, or incorporating strength training exercises into our fitness regimen, staying active is crucial for our overall health.

Nutrition and healthy eating go hand in hand with physical fitness. As adults, we must pay close attention to the food we consume, ensuring it is nourishing and beneficial for our bodies. A balanced diet rich in fruits, vegetables, whole grains, lean proteins, and healthy fats provides us with the necessary nutrients to fuel our bodies, boost our immune system, and prevent chronic diseases. By adopting mindful eating habits, such as portion control and reducing the intake of processed foods and sugary drinks, we can maintain a healthy weight and improve our overall well-being.

Weight loss and a healthy lifestyle should be approached with a long-term perspective. It is crucial to focus on sustainable lifestyle changes rather than quick fixes or fad diets. By setting realistic goals, creating a support system, and seeking professional guidance when needed, we can achieve and maintain a healthy weight. Remember, weight loss is not just about appearance but also about improving our overall health and reducing the risk of chronic diseases.

In conclusion, as adults, it is our responsibility to prioritize our physical fitness, nutrition, and overall well-being. By embracing a fit and healthy lifestyle, we can experience numerous benefits such as increased energy levels, improved mental well-being, and reduced risk of chronic diseases. Let "Fit for Life: The Ultimate Guide to Physical Fitness and Exercise for Adults" serve as a comprehensive resource to support and guide you on your journey towards a healthier and happier adulthood. Remember, it's never too late to start, and every small step towards a healthier lifestyle counts. Embrace the power of a fit and healthy life and unlock your true potential!